The diabetes protocol:

How to naturally prevent and treat type 2 diabetes

By

Victoria Elias

Table of contents

Chapter 1

What is Diabetes

Diabetes is a chronic medical condition that makes it difficult for your body to regulate blood sugar (glucose) levels. Type 1 diabetes, an autoimmune disorder in which the body stops producing insulin, and type 2 diabetes, which develops when the body stops producing insulin or produces insufficient amounts of it, are the two main forms.

To maintain blood sugar levels under control and avoid issues, proper management is crucial. It's critical to get medical counsel for a diagnosis and treatment if you think you may have diabetes.

Diabetes types

The three primary kinds of diabetes are as follows:

1. Type 1 diabetes: In this kind, the pancreatic beta cells that produce insulin are wrongly attacked and destroyed by the immune system. High blood sugar levels come from the pancreas producing little to no insulin. Typically, type 1 diabetes is discovered in children and young adults, and insulin therapy is necessary for effective care.

2. Type 2 Diabetes: Insulin resistance is a feature of type 2 diabetes, which is the most prevalent type. It happens when the body's cells do not respond to insulin as well as they should, and the pancreas may not generate enough insulin to offset the resistance. Obesity, inactivity, and bad eating patterns are among lifestyle variables that are frequently connected to type 2 diabetes. It can be controlled with medication, dietary adjustments, and occasionally insulin therapy.

3. Gestational Diabetes: Some pregnant women who did not previously have diabetes develop it during pregnancy. Insulin resistance can be brought on by hormonal changes during pregnancy. After giving delivery, gestational diabetes typically goes away, but it raises the chance of type 2 diabetes later in life.

Each type of diabetes has a unique management strategy, therefore it's critical for people with diabetes to collaborate closely with medical specialists to create an effective treatment regimen.

Diabetes causes

Depending on the kind, many factors might cause diabetes:

1. Type 1 diabetes: Although the exact cause is unknown, it is thought to be an autoimmune reaction in which the body's immune system targets and kills the cells that make insulin in the pancreas. Environmental elements and genetic predisposition might both be important.

2. Type 2 diabetes: This form is closely linked to bad eating patterns, inactivity, and lifestyle variables such being overweight or obese. The development of it may also be influenced by genetic factors. When the body develops an insulin resistance and the pancreas is unable to produce enough insulin to make up for it, type 2 diabetes results.

Age, ethnicity, having gestational diabetes while pregnant, and several medical disorders are additional factors that may raise the risk of acquiring diabetes.

Keep in mind that diabetes is a complicated disorder with a range of possible causes. Consult a healthcare expert if you are concerned about diabetes for an accurate assessment and recommendations.

Chapter 2

How type 2 diabetes spread to epidemic levels

A number of connected factors, including dietary and lifestyle changes as well as population aging, contributed to the emergence of the type 2 diabetes epidemic. Insulin resistance, a key risk factor for type 2 diabetes, has increased as a result of sedentary lifestyles, poor dietary practices, and rising obesity rates. The prevalence of the disease is also influenced by genetic predisposition and environmental factors. Numerous studies have been conducted and initiatives to promote diabetes prevention and improved management have been made as a result of the condition's rising prevalence becoming a serious public health concern.

Certainly! Let's examine the causes of the outbreak of type 2 diabetes in more detail:

1. Lifestyle Changes: Due to urbanization and technological improvements, many people now lead more sedentary lifestyles. The

fall in energy expenditure brought on by the decline in physical activity and the rise in sitting time has facilitated weight gain and obesity. Regular physical activity is crucial for preserving optimal insulin sensitivity, and a lack of it has elevated the risk of type 2 diabetes.

2. Dietary Habits: A rise in the consumption of processed and sugary foods, calorie-dense beverages, and fast food has been a hallmark of changes in dietary habits, notably in Western nations and metropolitan regions. These diets, which are frequently high in

unhealthy fats and processed carbs, can cause weight gain and insulin resistance, two major risk factors for type 2 diabetes.

3. Obesity: The epidemic of type 2 diabetes has been greatly aided by the global rise in obesity rates. Increased risk of developing diabetes and insulin resistance are both highly correlated with excess body fat, particularly around the belly. Obesity is one of the main risk factors for the condition, according to the World Health Organization (WHO).

4. Aging Population: Type 2 diabetes has become more common as the world's population has gotten older. Elderly people are more prone to both insulin resistance and reduced glucose tolerance, which increases their risk of developing the disorder.

5. Genetic Predisposition: Type 2 diabetes can also be influenced by a person's genes. The disease is more genetically predisposed to certain racial and ethnic groupings. The rising prevalence, however, cannot be simply attributable to genetics

because lifestyle choices have a big impact on how it develops.

6. Urbanization and Globalization: In many societies, rapid urbanization and globalization have altered conventional food and physical activity patterns. Urban locations frequently experience difficulties with regard to obtaining nutritious foods, having fewer opportunities for physical activity, and being more exposed to obesogenic settings.

7. Inadequate Awareness and Early Detection: In some areas, a lack of knowledge of diabetes, its risk

factors, and symptoms leads to a delayed diagnosis and subpar disease treatment. The burden of the disease can rise and serious complications as a result of delayed detection.

8. Inadequate healthcare access and infrastructure in some areas can make it difficult to diagnose diabetes early and treat it well, which has a negative impact on patient outcomes. A multipronged strategy is needed to combat the type 2 diabetes epidemic, including public health initiatives aimed at encouraging healthy eating, improving dietary practices,

increasing physical activity, and improving healthcare infrastructure to ensure early detection and efficient management of the condition. In order to prevent the chronic disease's increased prevalence, education and awareness initiatives are essential.

Chapter 3

Type 1 and Type 2 Diabetes: Differences

Diabetes comes in two different forms: type 1 and type 2, each of which has its own causes, traits, and methods of treatment. Effective management and prevention of these two illnesses depend on having a clear understanding of their differences. The causes, onset ages, treatments, and long-term effects of type 1 and type 2 diabetes will all be covered in this thorough overview.

Definition and root

In type 1 diabetes, also known as insulin-dependent diabetes or juvenile diabetes, the immune system mistakenly targets and kills the insulin-producing beta cells in the pancreas.

Because of this, those who have type 1 diabetes seldom or never produce insulin, a hormone that controls blood sugar levels. Type 1 diabetes is thought to be brought on by a confluence of genetic predisposition and environmental triggers, such as viral infections, however its specific etiology is yet unknown.

Contrarily, insulin resistance is the main feature of type 2 diabetes, also referred to as adult-onset diabetes. When the body's cells are unable to utilize insulin properly, this condition develops, and the pancreas may not generate enough insulin to make up for it. Obesity, bad eating habits, and sedentary activity are among lifestyle variables that are frequently linked to type 2 diabetes. Family history is a risk factor for type 2 diabetes, which is also greatly influenced by genetics.

The age of onset is:
The age at which type 1 and type 2 diabetes first appear is one of their main distinctions. Although it can happen at any age, type 1 diabetes commonly occurs in children, teenagers, or young adults. It frequently starts very quickly, and symptoms might strike out of nowhere. Type 2 diabetes, in contrast, typically affects adults over the age of 40. However, type 2 diabetes is increasingly being

identified in children and teenagers due to the growth in childhood obesity and sedentary lifestyles.

Glucose Dependence:

Another important distinction between type 1 and type 2 diabetes is the need for insulin. In type 1 diabetes, the loss of beta cells causes a complete lack of insulin. As a result, type 1 diabetics require ongoing insulin therapy via injections or insulin pumps to successfully control their blood sugar levels. Contrarily, type 2 diabetes is first controlled by making lifestyle adjustments such as eating a balanced diet and exercising frequently. To increase insulin sensitivity and glucose regulation, doctors may also prescribe oral medicines and non-insulin injectable drugs. To maintain healthy blood sugar levels, some type 2 diabetics may eventually need insulin therapy as their disease worsens.

Body mass index and obesity:
An essential contrast between the two forms of diabetes is how they relate to body weight and obesity. Type 2 diabetes is intimately linked to excess body weight, especially abdominal obesity, but type 1

diabetes is unrelated to body weight or obesity. Although obesity is a major risk factor for type 2 diabetes, not everyone who has the disease is overweight or obese.

Disease Progression:

Another distinction between type 1 and type 2 diabetes is how the disease develops over time. When type 1 diabetes is present, symptoms frequently occur unexpectedly and acutely. Diabetic ketoacidosis (DKA), a potentially fatal disease, can occur in people with type 1 diabetes if it is not managed. When the body breaks down fat for energy, acidic ketones are produced, which can be dangerous in excessive doses. On the other hand, type 2 diabetes frequently takes time to develop, and the early stages may not show as many symptoms. As type 2 diabetes worsens, people may get increased thirst, frequent urination, exhaustion, and blurred vision. Sometimes a gradual onset of symptoms can result in a delayed diagnosis and course of treatment.

Prevention

Because type 1 and type 2 diabetes have different underlying causes, their prevention techniques are also different. Unfortunately, type 1 diabetes cannot be prevented because its underlying cause cannot be avoided. The cause of type 1 diabetes is assumed to be a confluence of uncontrollable environmental stimuli and genetic predisposition. On the other hand, by managing risk factors and altering lifestyle, many occurrences of type 2 diabetes can be avoided or postponed. A balanced diet, frequent physical activity, and maintaining a healthy weight are all important factors in lowering the risk of developing type 2 diabetes. Early detection and care can dramatically lower the risk of developing type 2 diabetes, especially in people with prediabetes (a condition in which blood sugar levels are higher than normal but not high enough for a diabetes diagnosis).

Treatment and administration

Based on the underlying mechanisms and causes of type 1 and type 2 diabetes, different treatment strategies are used.

Insulin therapy is the mainstay of care for type 1 diabetes. For several daily insulin injections or continuous insulin delivery throughout the day, type 1 diabetics use insulin pumps. For the purpose of modifying insulin dosages and preserving stable glucose levels, frequent blood sugar monitoring is crucial. Devices for continuous glucose monitoring (CGM) have grown in popularity because they allow for more accurate and immediate monitoring. Changes in lifestyle are essential in the initial management of type 2 diabetes. Adopting a nutritious diet, getting regular exercise, and keeping a healthy weight are a few of these adjustments. To increase insulin sensitivity, boost insulin production, or lessen liver glucose production, doctors may give oral medicines. Non-insulin injectable drugs, like SGLT2 inhibitors and GLP-1 receptor agonists, have also shown promise in the treatment of type 2 diabetes. As their condition worsens, some persons with type 2 diabetes may require insulin therapy to get the best blood sugar control. In contrast to type 1 diabetes, type 2 diabetes is treated with insulin treatment, which augments rather than completely replaces the body's production of insulin.

Long-term issues include:
If not treated properly, both type 1 and type 2 diabetes can result in serious long-term problems. The risk of different issues affecting the eyes, kidneys, heart, and nerves increases when blood sugar levels in the body rise over time.
This can also cause damage to blood vessels and neurons.

Diabetic retinopathy, a major contributor to blindness, diabetic nephropathy, diabetic neuropathy, and an elevated risk of cardiovascular disorders like heart attacks and strokes are some of the long-term effects of diabetes.

Strict blood sugar management is essential in preventing or delaying the onset of these consequences, as well as routine medical exams and comprehensive diabetes care. In conclusion, type 1 diabetes and type 2 diabetes are two separate types of the disease with differing etiologies, ages of onset, insulin reliance, relationships with body weight, progression patterns, and therapeutic modalities. Type 2 diabetes largely involves insulin resistance and is frequently linked to lifestyle factors and genetics, whereas type 1 diabetes is an autoimmune illness defined by the loss of insulin-producing beta cells. In order to properly manage and prevent diabetes, healthcare professionals, patients, and the general public must all be aware of these disparities. Diabetes and its complications place a heavy cost on people and healthcare systems around the world. Reducing this burden requires early diagnosis, appropriate treatment, and adherence to healthy lifestyle behaviors. The quality of life for persons affected by these illnesses is also continuing to improve because of ongoing research and breakthroughs in diabetes care.

Chapter 4

The overall impact on the body

Diabetes is a long-term metabolic illness that impairs the body's capacity to maintain healthy blood sugar levels. Over time, having high blood sugar levels can cause a number of issues that affect different organ systems. In this thorough overview, we'll examine the impact of diabetes on several physiological systems and the significance of effective management to avert or postpone these issues.

Included in the cardiovascular system are:

Cardiovascular disease risk is greatly increased by diabetes. As a result of atherosclerosis, which occurs when fatty deposits accumulate in the arteries and restrict them and block blood flow, high blood sugar levels can harm blood vessels. Peripheral artery disease, strokes, and heart attacks are all made more likely by this illness. Diabetes can also result in blood lipid abnormalities and hypertension (high blood pressure), which raises cardiovascular risk even further.

Nervous System:

Diabetes frequently results in diabetic neuropathy, which damages the nerves, especially in the extremities. The hands and feet may experience tingling, numbness, burning, or pain as symptoms. This illness has the potential to cause sensory loss over time, making it challenging for sufferers to detect injuries or infections in their limbs. When neuropathy is severe, internal organs might also be affected, which can cause gastrointestinal problems and sexual dysfunction.

Vision and the Eyes:

Adult blindness is most frequently caused by diabetic retinopathy. If untreated, high blood sugar damages the retina's blood vessels, resulting in visual issues and even blindness. Further affecting eyesight, diabetes also ups the risk of glaucoma and cataracts.

The kidneys:

Diabetes-related kidney disease is known as diabetic nephropathy. High blood sugar levels can harm the kidneys' teeny blood vessels, making it harder for them to adequately filter toxins and waste from the blood. It can develop into end-stage kidney disease, necessitating dialysis or kidney transplantation, if neglected.

Skin and Wound Recovery:

Diabetes patients are more likely to have skin problems because of impaired nerve function and decreased blood flow. Even small wounds can result in dangerous infections and take longer to heal than minor cuts, blisters, or sores. Dry, itchy skin is also a result of poor circulation, and diabetic foot ulcers are a major worry.

Immune System:

Diabetes can impair immunological function, increasing a person's susceptibility to infections. Skin infections, urinary tract infections, and problems with oral health are all made more likely by high blood sugar levels, which create an ideal habitat for bacteria and fungi to flourish.

The reproductive system

Both men and women who have uncontrolled diabetes can experience issues with their reproductive systems. Diabetes can cause erectile dysfunction in males by damaging blood vessels and nerves. Diabetes can cause irregular menstrual periods in women and increase their risk of miscarriage, urinary tract infections, and miscarriage.

The digestive system:
The digestive system can be impacted by diabetes, which can result in problems like gastroparesis, a disease where the stomach takes longer to empty its contents. Symptoms including bloating, nausea, and vomiting may result from this. Additionally, diabetes can harm the nerves that manage the lower digestive system, resulting in diarrhea or constipation.

Bone Health:

According to recent research, diabetes may have an impact on bone health, raising the risk of fractures and osteoporosis. In people with diabetes, decreased bone production and increased bone resorption may contribute to changes in bone density and strength.

Mental Wellness:

Mental health can be significantly impacted by having diabetes. Stress, worry, and sadness might result from the ongoing need for self-management, blood sugar monitoring, and potential problems. To cope effectively, people with diabetes need enough emotional support and access to mental health care.

A disorder with many facets and complexity, diabetes can have an impact on almost every organ system in the body. Diabetes's high blood sugar levels can cause a variety of complications, including kidney damage, skin difficulties, visual troubles, neuropathy, cardiovascular disorders, and neuropathy.

The start of these consequences can be delayed or avoided with proper diabetes treatment, which includes regular blood sugar testing, medication adherence, lifestyle changes, and regular medical checkups. Working together with medical providers to create a thorough management plan customized to their unique needs and medical background is vital for people with diabetes. The quality of life for persons with diabetes can be greatly enhanced, and the chance of complications that may have an effect on the body as a whole can be decreased, with the help of medical care, good lifestyle choices, and emotional support. Additional prospects for better outcomes and better management of this chronic condition are always being presented by continuing research and medical developments in the field of diabetes treatment.

Chapter 5

Diabetes: a lie in the media

The notion that all calories are the same and that counting calories is the only method of managing diabetes is referred to as the "calorie deception". However, this viewpoint oversimplifies the intricate connection between calories, controlling blood sugar levels, and general health for those with diabetes. In this discussion, we'll look at the calorie illusion, its effects on managing diabetes, and the significance of taking into account more than just calories. Caloric Intake and Blood Sugar Calories, a unit of measurement for food energy, are important for controlling blood sugar levels. Our diet's main sources of calories are proteins, lipids, and carbs. Sugars and starches in particular, which are converted down into glucose during digestion, have the greatest immediate effect on blood sugar levels of all the carbohydrates. For diabetics, controlling calorie consumption is crucial, especially for those attempting to maintain a healthy weight. No matter where they come from, consuming too many calories can cause weight gain and aggravate insulin resistance in people with type 2 diabetes. On the other hand, malnutrition and insufficient energy levels can result from continuously consuming too little calories.

Calorie Quality

The value of consuming high-quality calories is sometimes overlooked by the calorie trick. Regarding their nutritional content and effects on general health, not all calories are created equal. For instance, 100 calories from a sugary soft drink would differ from 100 calories from nutrient-rich fruits or vegetables in terms of how they affect blood sugar levels and general health. Making healthy food choices that are complete, unprocessed, and high in fiber, vitamins, and minerals can help to maintain stable blood sugar levels. Foods that are high in nutrients are advantageous for diabetics since they offer vital nutrients while limiting calories.

The glycemic index and load are three.
The glycemic index (GI) measures carbohydrates according to how rapidly they cause blood sugar levels to rise upon eating. While foods with a high GI quickly raise

blood sugar levels, those with a low GI do so gradually. People with diabetes may find it useful to take the GI of foods into account while managing their blood sugar levels. The quantity and type of carbohydrates in a food are both taken into account by the glycemic load (GL). Compared to focusing only on the GI, it offers a more realistic picture of how a specific food will impact blood sugar levels.

Insulin Response

The calorie trick ignores the significance of the body's insulin reaction to various foods. By making it easier for glucose to enter cells for use as fuel or storage, the hormone insulin aids in controlling blood sugar levels. Proteins and lipids have a softer impact on insulin release than carbohydrates. Even if their overall caloric consumption is within control, some diabetics may experience higher blood sugar increases after eating meals high in carbohydrates. Understanding how each person's body reacts to various foods might help you make better dietary decisions and regulate your blood sugar levels.

Individual Differences

Since every diabetic is different, so might be how they react to certain meals and calories. The body's ability to digest calories and control blood sugar is influenced by factors like insulin sensitivity, medication use, physical activity, and metabolism. For some people with diabetes, the "one-size-fits-all" method of calorie counting may not be appropriate.

Emotional and social factors

Beyond calorie counting, managing diabetes also entails taking social and emotional issues into account. Blood sugar levels and dietary preferences can be affected by stress, emotional eating, and social circumstances. Support networks and emotional well-being are essential elements of successful diabetes control.

Weight Management and Loss

Weight loss can considerably increase insulin sensitivity and blood sugar control in people with type 2 diabetes who are overweight or obese. However, cutting calories shouldn't be the only thing on your mind. The easiest way to lose weight permanently is to combine a balanced diet with more exercise and change your habits.

Education about nutrition

It's crucial to encourage a deeper comprehension of nutrition and how it affects the control of diabetes. The significance of maintaining a macronutrient balance, selecting wholesome foods, and taking into account how different foods may affect different people should all be emphasized in nutritional education. The dangers of excessive dietary restrictions and the significance of fulfilling nutritional needs for critical nutrients should also be covered.

The calorie misconception oversimplifies how calories relate to managing diabetes. While calorie consumption is crucial, it is also necessary to take into account food's overall nutritional value, glycemic index, glycemic load, and individual insulin responses. Beyond calorie tracking, managing diabetes requires a holistic strategy that takes into account emotional, social, and physical components. Individualized nutrition programs, routine blood sugar testing, and an emphasis on nutrient-dense, whole foods can help people with diabetes maintain stable blood sugar levels and improve their general health. Personalized and sustainable dietary strategies are essential for helping people with diabetes thrive and lower the risk of complications. Dietitians and diabetes educators should work together with other healthcare professionals to design these strategies. Beyond calorie counting, a holistic approach to diabetes care takes into account the complex interplay of numerous elements that improve overall wellbeing and the course of diabetes.

Chapter 6

Insulin's involvement in energy storage

Insulin is essential for energy storage in the human body. It is a pancreatic hormone that regulates blood glucose levels and influences the storage and utilization of nutrients, notably carbohydrates and lipids. In this discussion, we will look at insulin's diverse involvement in energy storage, from secretion and action to its effects on various tissues and organs.

Secretion of Insulin

Insulin is created and released by beta cells, which are specialized cells in the pancreas. When blood sugar levels rise after eating, the pancreas senses it and responds by releasing insulin into the bloodstream. The primary stimulus for insulin secretion is an increase in blood glucose, though amino acids and gastrointestinal hormones can also cause insulin release.

Insulin Receptors and Signaling

Insulin interacts with specific receptors on the surface of target cells after being released into the bloodstream, triggering a series of chemical events known as insulin signaling. The insulin receptor is a protein that spans the cell membrane and when activated by insulin, it initiates intracellular signaling pathways.

Muscle and Adipose Tissue Glucose UptakeEnhancing glucose absorption by muscle and adipose (fat) tissue is one of insulin's main roles.Insulin stimulates the translocation of glucose transporter

proteins, particularly GLUT4, to the cell membrane in skeletal muscle cells. This lets glucose reach muscle cells, where it can be stored as glycogen or utilized to produce energy. Insulin increases glucose absorption and conversion into fatty acids in adipose tissue, which are then deposited as triglycerides in fat cells.

Liver and Muscle Glycogen Synthesis

Insulin is essential for glycogen synthesis, which is the process by which excess glucose is turned into glycogen for storage. Insulin increases glucose uptake and glycogen conversion in the liver, which helps to reduce blood glucose levels. Similarly, insulin stimulates the creation of glycogen in skeletal muscle cells, which can be used as an energy store for muscle activity.

Glucose Production Inhibition

Insulin inhibits hepatic gluconeogenesis, or the generation of glucose in the liver. Insulin helps prevent excessive glucose release into the bloodstream by preventing the creation of new glucose molecules from non-carbohydrate sources, keeping blood sugar within a safe range.

Adipose Tissue and Lipid Metabolism

Insulin also has an impact on lipid (fat) metabolism. Insulin increases the uptake of fatty acids and glucose in adipose tissue, where they are mixed to produce triglycerides. These triglycerides are deposited within fat cells as fat droplets. Insulin also slows lipolysis, the breakdown of stored triglycerides into fatty acids, lowering fatty acid release into the bloodstream.

Protein Synthesis and Amino Acid Absorption

Insulin stimulates the uptake of amino acids into muscle cells, which aids in protein synthesis. It improves the transport of amino acids across cell membranes, supplying the building blocks required for protein synthesis and repair. This is especially necessary after eating to promote tissue growth and repair.

Importance in Energy Homeostasis

Insulin is an important regulator of energy homeostasis, which is a careful balance of energy intake, storage, and utilization. When blood sugar levels rise after a meal, insulin aids in the storage of extra nutrients as glycogen in the liver and muscles and fat in adipose tissue. Insulin levels fall between meals or during fasting periods, allowing the body to use stored energy stores to meet its energy needs.

Brain Function

Insulin also has a role in the brain, acting as a neurotransmitter. It has an impact on brain functions such as hunger management, cognition, and memory.

Brain insulin signaling dysfunction has been linked to

neurodegenerative diseases such as Alzheimer's.

Feedback Mechanisms for Regulation

To keep blood sugar levels within a small range, feedback systems closely regulate insulin output. Following a meal, insulin is produced to enhance glucose uptake and storage. As blood glucose levels fall, so does insulin release, allowing the body to draw on stored energy reserves.

Diabetes Dysregulation

Diabetes impairs insulin's normal function, resulting in blood sugar dysregulation and energy storage. The immune system targets and destroys the insulin-producing beta cells in the pancreas in type 1 diabetes, resulting in little or no insulin production. Individuals with type 1 diabetes require insulin therapy for the rest of their lives to control their blood sugar levels.

The body develops resistance to the effects of insulin in type 2 diabetes, and the pancreas may not generate enough insulin to compensate. Insulin resistance reduces glucose uptake in muscle and adipose tissue, resulting in high blood sugar levels. The pancreas may struggle to maintain enough insulin secretion over time, causing persistent hyperglycemia.

Diabetes Management Implication

Understanding insulin's role in energy storage is critical for diabetic management. Insulin therapy is a critical component of treatment for people with type 1 diabetes. They can manage blood sugar levels and facilitate energy storage in the form of glycogen and fat by providing insulin via injections or insulin pumps.

To enhance insulin sensitivity in people with type 2 diabetes, lifestyle changes such as a balanced diet, regular physical activity, and weight management are essential. To achieve optimal blood sugar control, medications that improve insulin action or promote insulin production may be recommended.

Insulin is important for energy storage in the body because it facilitates glucose uptake in muscle and adipose tissue, promotes glycogen synthesis in the liver and muscles, inhibits glucose production in the liver, and influences lipid and protein metabolism. It is an important regulator of energy homeostasis, keeping blood sugar levels within a limited range. If left untreated, insulin dysregulation in diabetes can result in high blood sugar levels and consequences. Understanding insulin's varied role in diabetes management is critical for helping people with diabetes achieve better blood sugar control and overall health.

Diabetes mellitus and insulin resistanc

When the body's cells cease reacting to the effects of insulin, which results in a spike in blood sugar levels, this metabolic disease is known as insulin resistance. The cycle of glucose and fatty acids, also known as the overflow phenomenon, is one of the processes that results in insulin resistance. In this talk, we will go through insulin resistance, the overflow phenomenon, how it affects the metabolism of glucose and fatty acids, and how it affects overall health.

Recognizing Insulin Resistance

Insulin, a hormone secreted by the pancreas, is crucial for regulating blood sugar levels. Insulin is released to aid in the absorption of glucose into cells, where it can be utilized for energy or stored as glycogen, as blood sugar levels rise after a meal. Additionally, insulin prevents the liver from releasing glucose, which aids in maintaining steady blood sugar levels between meals. When cells in the body, such as those in the muscle, liver, and adipose tissue, lose their sensitivity to the effects of insulin, this condition is known as insulin resistance. As a result, the body needs more insulin to achieve the same levels of glucose absorption and storage, which raises blood sugar levels. If left untreated, this disease might eventually lead to prediabetes and type 2 diabetes.

Contributing factors for insulin resistance include:

Insulin resistance is a complicated condition that is affected by a number of variables:

1: Obesity

Insulin resistance is linked to extra adipose tissue, particularly visceral fat (fat accumulated around internal organs). Inflammatory substances generated by adipose tissue disrupt insulin signaling in other tissues.

2: Physical Irregularity

Regular exercise increases insulin sensitivity, but inactivity increases insulin resistance.

3: Genetics

Some people are genetically predisposed to insulin resistance, which increases their risk of type 2 diabetes.

4: Inflammation Insulin resistance and persistent low-grade inflammation are related.

Inflammatory substances can obstruct the pathways that insulin uses for signaling.

5: Dietary factors include: Insulin resistance can be exacerbated by a diet high in processed carbs, added sugars, and unhealthy fats.

6: Hormones are: several hormones, including the stress hormone cortisol and several sex hormones, might affect insulin sensitivity.

7: Age Because insulin sensitivity tends to decline with age, older people are more likely to develop insulin resistance.

The Overflow Phenomenon

One of the mechanisms that helps explain insulin resistance is the overflow phenomenon, often known as the glucose-fatty acid cycle. In response to insulin resistance, both glucose and fatty acids are simultaneously released into the bloodstream. Adipose tissue and the liver are where this phenomena mostly occurs.

Fatty Acid Release from Adipose Tissue:

The regular control of lipolysis, which is the conversion of triglycerides stored in adipose tissue into fatty acids, is thrown off in insulin-resistant adipose tissue. Fatty acids are consequently released into the bloodstream at a higher rate. These extra fatty acids can worsen insulin signaling in muscle and liver cells, which can further contribute to insulin resistance.

Liver's Function in the Overflow Phenomenon

Insulin often inhibits gluconeogenesis, the process of producing glucose from non-carbohydrate sources including amino acids and fatty acids, in the liver. Because the liver is less sensitive to the inhibitory effects of insulin, there is more glucose produced and released into the bloodstream when there is insulin resistance. In turn, this causes blood sugar levels to increase.

Effects on the Metabolism of Glucose

Several factors in the overflow phenomena cause blood sugar levels to rise:

1: Lower Glucose Uptake: The amount of glucose that is delivered from the bloodstream into muscle cells for energy or glycogen storage is decreased due to insulin resistance in muscle cells.

2: The production of glucose has increased. Increased gluconeogenesis, which results in higher glucose production and release into the bloodstream, is made possible by insulin resistance in the liver.

3: Improved glucose release from adipose tissue:

The Randle cycle, often referred to as the glucose-fatty acid cycle, is a mechanism by which fatty acids produced from insulin-resistant adipose tissue can increase glucose synthesis in the liver. This causes the blood sugar levels to rise even more.

Effects on the Metabolism of Fatty Acids

The overflow phenomenon affects fatty acid metabolism as well:

1: Enhanced Fatty Acid Release The development of ectopic fat accumulation may be facilitated by the release of extra fatty acids from adipose tissue that is resistant to insulin. Ectopic fat is the term used to describe the deposit of fat in non-adipose tissues such the pancreas, liver, and muscles.

2: Increased lipotoxicity: Lipotoxicity can result from the buildup of extra fatty acids in tissues other than adipose tissue. High quantities of fatty acids can have detrimental effects on cellular activity and insulin sensitivity, a condition known as lipotoxicity. It aids in the growth of type 2 diabetes and the advancement of insulin resistance.

Consequences for Overall Health:

The overflow phenomenon and insulin resistance have significant effects on general health:

1: Diabetes type 2: Insulin resistance that persists can cause poor glucose regulation and the onset of type 2 diabetes. Over time, high blood sugar levels can harm organs, blood vessels, and nerves, which can result in a number of issues connected to diabetes.

2: Heart and Vascular Health: Heart attacks and strokes are among the cardiovascular disorders that are intimately linked to insulin resistance. Excess fatty acids and elevated blood sugar levels have the potential to accelerate atherosclerosis and blood vessel inflammation.

3 Fat Liver Disorder: Non-alcoholic fatty liver disease (NAFLD) is a condition whose development is influenced by the overflow phenomena. If unchecked, liver fat accumulation can lead to cirrhosis, fibrosis, and non-alcoholic steatohepatitis (NASH).

4: Obesity: A vicious cycle results when insulin resistance and the overflow phenomenon make obesity worse, and obesity then makes insulin resistance worse.

5: Inflammation Increased inflammation in many tissues brought on by the overflow phenomena and ectopic fat buildup can aid in the onset of chronic illness.

Chapter 8

Fructose's connection to insulin resistance

Research on and discussion of fructose's potential connection to insulin resistance have increased recently. I will discuss the impacts of fructose on metabolism, potential processes, and health consequences in this response, which will be about 1000 words long.

A disease known as insulin resistance occurs when the body's cells stop responding to the hormone insulin, which the pancreas produces and uses to help control blood sugar levels. Elevated blood sugar levels result from cells that are insulin resistant that have trouble absorbing glucose from the bloodstream. This syndrome has the potential to develop into type 2 diabetes and other metabolic disorders over time. A natural simple sugar called fructose can be found in various fruits, honey, and vegetables. It is also a key ingredient in high-fructose corn syrup (HFCS), a common sweetener found in processed foods and beverages, as well as table sugar (sucrose). Fructose is largely digested in the liver, as opposed to glucose, which is generally done so by every cell in the body.

The liver starts the process of breaking down fructose into fructose-1-phosphate, which is then further broken down into intermediate metabolites such glyceraldehyde and dihydroxyacetone phosphate. These intermediates can enter a number of metabolic processes that produce fatty acids, glucose, and glycogen.

The potential for increased fructose consumption to increase insulin resistance is one of the main issues. Excessive fructose consumption has been linked to insulin resistance in a number of ways, including the following:

1. Increased Fat Accumulation: Fructose metabolism in the liver results in an increase in fatty acid and triglyceride production. Overloading the liver's ability to store fat can cause non-alcoholic fatty liver disease (NAFLD), which is characterized by an accumulation of fat in the liver cells. Insulin resistance has been connected to the increased liver fat.

2. Impaired Insulin Signaling: Consuming fructose has been found to interfere with the routes that insulin uses to communicate with cells, reducing insulin sensitivity. As a result, insulin is less effective at encouraging the uptake of glucose by cells, raising blood sugar levels.

3. Increased Inflammation: Regularly consuming high fructose meals may cause the body to become more inflamed. Because it interferes with insulin signaling and damages cellular function, inflammation can increase the risk of developing insulin resistance.

4. Modified Gut Microbiota: According to certain research, high fructose consumption may result in modifications to the composition of the gut microbiota. Insulin resistance may result from an unbalanced gut bacterial population that affects metabolism and inflammation.

Cellular metabolism of fructose can also result in the creation of ROS. ROS are chemicals that have the potential to harm cellular architecture and increase insulin resistance. It is important to understand that the relationship between fructose consumption and insulin resistance is complicated and may differ depending on a number of variables, including total calorie intake, the overall quality of the diet, and certain metabolic traits.

Furthermore, not every study yields reliable conclusions, and some studies suggest that moderate fructose intake from natural sources, such as whole fruits, may not have the same adverse consequences as excessive consumption of added sugars or high-fructose corn syrup found in processed foods.

The American Heart Association (AHA) advises men and women to limit their daily intake of added sugar to 150 calories (about 9 teaspoons) for men and 100 calories (roughly 6 teaspoons) for women. Concerns regarding excessive fructose consumption and its potential consequences on metabolic health are addressed by these recommendations. Overall, it is important to keep in mind that a well-balanced diet high in whole foods and low in added sugars is crucial for maintaining overall health and preventing chronic diseases, even though excessive fructose intake has been linked in some studies to insulin resistance and other metabolic problems. In conclusion, the relationship between fructose and insulin resistance is a complicated one with many facets. Consuming too much fructose, especially from added sugars and high-fructose corn syrup found in processed foods, may cause insulin resistance through a number of different mechanisms, including an increase in liver fat accumulation, impaired insulin signaling, inflammation, changes in the gut microbiota, and the production of ROS. However, more investigation is required to better comprehend the part fructose plays in insulin resistance and to pinpoint mitigation techniques for any potential negative effects. Like with every area of nutrition, promoting overall health and wellbeing requires moderation and a balanced diet.

Chapter 9

Metabolic syndrome and diabetes

Diabetes and metabolic syndrome are closely related diseases with similar underlying causes and risk factors. A group of related risk factors known as metabolic syndrome raises the possibility of getting type 2 diabetes, cardiovascular disease, and other illnesses. I'll explain how the metabolic syndrome and diabetes are related in this answer. The term "metabolic syndrome" refers to a collection of related illnesses rather than a single disease, such as:

1.1. Insulin Resistance: Insulin resistance is a feature of metabolic syndrome. It makes reference to how cells' impaired ability to adequately respond to insulin results in an increase in blood sugar levels.Hyperinsulinemia (high insulin levels in the blood) can occur as a result of the pancreas producing more insulin when insulin resistance worsens.

2. Abdominal Obesity: Central obesity, often known as abdominal obesity, is characterized by an accumulation of extra fat around the waist. An higher risk of insulin resistance and several metabolic disorders are linked to this type of fat distribution.

3. Dyslipidemia: Abnormally high levels of lipids (such as cholesterol and triglycerides) in the blood are referred to as dyslipidemia. Increases in triglycerides, low-density lipoprotein (LDL) cholesterol (the "bad" cholesterol), and high-density lipoprotein (HDL) cholesterol (the "good" cholesterol) are common in metabolic syndrome.

4. High Blood Pressure: Another element of the metabolic syndrome is hypertension, or high blood pressure. It increases the risk of heart disease and adds to the stress on the cardiovascular system.

5. Elevated Fasting Blood Sugar: Metabolic syndrome sufferers frequently have higher fasting blood sugar readings, which shows some degree of impaired glucose metabolism.

Metabolic syndrome is defined as three or more of these disorders present. Type 2 diabetes and other health issues, including metabolic syndrome, are more likely to arise.

Since insulin resistance is a key component of both metabolic syndrome and diabetes, these two diseases are closely related to one another. Higher blood sugar levels result from cells that are less able to absorb glucose from the bloodstream as a result of insulin resistance. Prediabetes or type 2 diabetes may eventually appear if the pancreas is unable to produce enough insulin to counteract insulin resistance over time. Due to the adverse environment for glucose regulation that is created by the combination of insulin resistance and other metabolic abnormalities, people with metabolic syndrome are more likely to develop diabetes. Additionally, both metabolic syndrome and type 2 diabetes have the characteristics of abdominal obesity and excessive liver fat deposition (non-alcoholic fatty liver disease).

Given that those with metabolic syndrome are five times more likely than those without the syndrome to develop type 2 diabetes, there is a major link between the two conditions. Additionally, the risk of cardiovascular disease and associated consequences is increased when both metabolic syndrome and diabetes are present.

There are significant overlaps in the prevention and management of metabolic syndrome and diabetes. Changing one's way of life is essential for lowering the risk of both diseases. These may consist of:

1. Weight management: Reducing abdominal obesity and maintaining a healthy weight can increase

insulin sensitivity and lower the risk of developing diabetes and the metabolic syndrome.

2. Balanced Diet: Both disorders can be prevented and managed by following a balanced diet that is high in whole foods, fruits, vegetables, and lean proteins and low in added sweets and saturated fats.

3. Exercise: Engaging in regular exercise can help prevent or manage metabolic syndrome and diabetes as well as increase insulin sensitivity.

4. Monitoring Blood Pressure and cholesterol Levels: It's crucial to regularly check and control blood pressure and cholesterol levels to avoid the cardiovascular consequences that might arise from both disorders.

5. Medication: For those with metabolic syndrome and diabetes, medication may occasionally be administered to control blood sugar, blood pressure, and cholesterol levels.

In conclusion, insulin resistance and other metabolic abnormalities are features of the metabolic syndrome and diabetes, two illnesses that are closely associated. In order to avoid and treat these disorders and lower the risk of complications, it is essential to address risk factors through lifestyle modifications and, if necessary, pharmaceutical management. For those with metabolic syndrome and diabetes, early detection and intervention are essential for improving overall health outcomes and quality of life.

Chapter 10

Insulin is not a treatment for type 2 diabetes.

The body's dysfunctional response to the hormone insulin, which is in charge of controlling blood glucose levels, characterizes type 2 diabetes, a complex metabolic condition. If left untreated, this condition, sometimes referred to as insulin resistance, causes increased blood sugar levels that could have harmful health effects. Examining a number of interconnected elements, such as basic physiological mechanisms, lifestyle decisions, and heredity, can help us understand why type 2 diabetes does not respond to insulin.

The emergence of type 2 diabetes is significantly influenced by genetic factors. A person's genetic makeup may predispose them to developing insulin resistance, which would compromise the insulin signaling pathway. Reduced insulin sensitivity results from these mutations, which have an impact on important elements of the insulin receptor and downstream signaling cascades. Furthermore, adipokines, cytokines, and other molecules that support insulin resistance can be produced in response to genetic factors. Major risk factors for type 2 diabetes include obesity and sedentary behavior. The release of pro-inflammatory chemicals and hormones from excess adipose tissue, particularly in the abdominal area, disrupts insulin signaling. Physical inactivity exacerbates insulin resistance since exercise improves insulin sensitivity and muscle cell absorption of glucose.

In addition, nutrition is a major factor in insulin resistance. Consuming meals high in calories but poor in nutrients, such as processed foods and sugary drinks, can increase the risk of obesity and insulin resistance. A diet high in refined carbs and saturated fats can cause lipid accumulation in the tissues, which can increase inflammation and insulin resistance. Insulin resistance is mostly a result of chronic inflammation. Adipose tissue and skeletal muscle tissues, for example, are affected by inflammatory cytokines' disruption of insulin signaling pathways and promotion of insulin resistance. Obesity and other metabolic diseases are frequently linked to this inflammation. Another element linked to insulin resistance is mitochondrial malfunction.

Defective mitochondria, which are responsible for generating energy in cells, can lead to the accumulation of reactive oxygen species (ROS) and reduced cellular activity.By interacting with insulin signaling pathways, ROS leads to insulin resistance.

Additionally, changes in the gut flora have been connected to insulin resistance. Increased intestinal permeability and the generation of pro-inflammatory compounds are two effects that can result from dysbiosis, an imbalance in the gut microbial community. Both systemic inflammation and insulin resistance are influenced by these elements. Hormonal abnormalities also contribute to insulin resistance in addition to these other variables. Cortisol, glucagon, and growth hormone are a few examples of hormones that can block the actions of insulin, causing blood sugar levels to rise. Insulin resistance can worsen the illness by affecting the pancreas's ability to secrete insulin. Because of how these factors interact, a vicious cycle develops in which the pancreas produces more insulin to counteract insulin resistance and high blood sugar levels. This increased need for insulin over time may result in decreased insulin secretion and exhausted beta cells, which ultimately result in type 2 diabetes.

Modifying one's lifestyle to adopt a balanced diet and participate in regular physical activity are among the treatment options for type 2 diabetes. Medications may also be recommended to increase insulin sensitivity or lessen the liver's ability to produce glucose. To effectively control blood sugar levels in extreme situations, insulin therapy may be required. In conclusion, type 2 diabetes not responding to insulin is a complex illness driven by genetic predisposition, lifestyle decisions, and a variety of physiological factors. For this common and dangerous metabolic condition, understanding these intricate relationships is crucial to creating more effective preventative and treatment plans.

Chapter 11

Hypoglycemic oral: No reaction

There are a number of causes for type 2 diabetes not responding to oral hypoglycemic medicines, which can be roughly divided into patient-related factors and medication-related issues. Let's examine some of the typical causes of this, shall we?

1. Insulin Resistance: Type 2 diabetes causes the body's cells to develop a resistance to insulin's effects, which reduces glucose uptake and raises blood sugar levels. Metformin and sulfonylureas are two examples of oral hypoglycemic medications that lower blood sugar levels through various processes. However, if insulin resistance is severe, these drugs might not be adequate to treat it.

2. Beta-Cell Dysfunction: People with type 2 diabetes may experience compromised beta cells or insufficient insulin production. Oral medicines that promote insulin production, such as sulfonylureas or meglitinides, may not be sufficient to lower blood sugar levels if beta-cell function is considerably impaired.

3. Inadequate Dosage: Different people respond differently to oral hypoglycemic medicines. The recommended dosage might not always be enough to achieve the required blood sugar management. The healthcare professional may need to change the dosage or add other medications in such circumstances.

4. Non adherence to medication: including irregular consumption of oral hypoglycemic medications, might result in insufficient blood sugar management. To get the best outcomes, patients must take their prescriptions exactly as directed.

5. Lifestyle variables: Diet and exercise are key components of type 2 diabetes management. The effects of oral hypoglycemic medications may be diminished if a person maintains their unhealthy diet and sedentary lifestyle.

6. Disease Progression: Type 2 diabetes is a chronic condition that worsens over time, making oral treatments less effective. Insulin treatment or other stronger medications can be required when the illness worsens.

7. Drug Interactions: Taking some medications concurrently can reduce the effectiveness of oral hypoglycemic treatments. For instance, some drugs, such as corticosteroids or diuretics, may increase blood sugar levels or lessen the effectiveness of oral diabetes treatments.

8. Individual Variations: Genetic differences and other personal characteristics can affect how each person reacts to medication. One person's solution could not have the same impact on another.

9. Coexisting Medical Conditions: Some illnesses, such as renal or liver disease, can interfere with the metabolism and clearance of oral hypoglycemic drugs, potentially lowering the effectiveness of these drugs.

Healthcare professionals may look at alternate treatments, such as different drug classes, injectable medicines such GLP-1 receptor agonists, or insulin therapy, when type 2 diabetes cannot be successfully controlled with oral hypoglycemic drugs. In order to achieve optimal blood sugar management and lower the risk of complications connected to diabetes, patients must have individualized treatment programs that take into account their particular medical history, lifestyle choices, and disease development.

Chapter 12

Exercise and a low-calorie diet are not the solution.

When type 2 diabetes does not react to low-calorie diets and exercise, managing the condition can be difficult and unpleasant. Understanding these characteristics is crucial for maximizing diabetes treatment because several reasons may be responsible for this lack of response. Here are several explanations as to why low-calorie diets and exercise may not be as effective for type 2 diabetes as anticipated:

1. Insulin Resistance: Despite weight loss and increased physical activity, the body's cells may occasionally continue to be resistant to insulin. Even when other components of metabolic health improve, insulin resistance can still exist.

2. Beta-Cell Dysfunction: Type 2 diabetes is characterized by a reduced ability of the beta cells in the pancreas to secrete insulin. Although modifying one's lifestyle can help control diabetes, if one's beta-cell function is seriously compromised, this may not be enough to get one's blood sugar levels back to normal.

3. Individual Variability: Genetic, metabolic, and underlying medical issues can all have a significant impact on how individuals respond to diet and exercise. To establish glycemic control, certain people may require more aggressive measures.

4. Weight Loss Plateau: Low-calorie eating plans and regular exercise can initially result in significant weight loss and better diabetes management. However, as time goes on, the rate of weight reduction may slow down or plateau, which may have an effect on controlling blood sugar.

5. Dietary Composition: Both the quantity and quality of a low-calorie diet are important. For the control of diabetes, nutrient-dense foods with the proper distribution of macronutrients must be prioritized.

6. Glycemic Load: Foods' glycemic loads can affect how much sugar is absorbed into the body. Even with a low-calorie diet, some meals that seem healthy might nevertheless produce large blood sugar rises.

7. Stress and Cortisol: Prolonged stress can raise cortisol levels, which may contradict the health benefits of lifestyle modifications.

8. Medication: Even with lifestyle changes, some people with type 2 diabetes may still need medication to achieve sufficient blood sugar management. Supplementing lifestyle changes with medications can help control the disease more successfully. Coexisting medical diseases might alter blood sugar levels and diabetes care, such as hormone imbalances or sleep disturbances.

9. Non-Adherence: To achieve the best results, a low-calorie diet and frequent exercise must be strictly followed. Progress may be hampered if the recommended routine is not followed.

10. Underlying Inflammation: Even with lifestyle modifications, chronic inflammation can increase insulin resistance and make it more difficult to treat diabetes.

Healthcare professionals may suggest further treatments, such as oral drugs, injectable therapies like GLP-1 receptor agonists or insulin, or other cutting-edge strategies, when lifestyle changes alone do not produce the desired results. Type 2 diabetes is managed with a customised strategy that considers unique health requirements and preferences. Finding the best methods to control diabetes and enhance general health outcomes can be facilitated by close collaboration with medical experts.

Chapter 13
Reduced-carbohydrate diet

A diet low in carbohydrates can be a successful and tried and true method for managing type 2 diabetes. This dietary approach focuses on lowering carbohydrate intake, especially those that spike blood sugar levels quickly, to help improve glycemic control and metabolic health in general. The main advantages and guidelines of a diet low in carbohydrates for the management of type 2 diabetes are as follows:

1. Better Blood Sugar Control: Blood sugar levels can be better managed by consuming fewer carbohydrates, especially simple sugars and refined carbohydrates. As a result, there may be less chance of experiencing episodes of hyperglycemia (high blood sugar) and hypoglycemia (low blood sugar).

2. Weight Management: Studies have shown that diets low in carbohydrates are useful for both

weight loss and weight management. Being a healthy weight and keeping it off are essential for managing type 2 diabetes because they can improve insulin sensitivity and lower insulin resistance.

3. Less Insulin Needed: The body may need less insulin to control blood sugar levels if there are fewer carbohydrates in the diet. This can result in more consistent insulin dose, which is advantageous for people with insulin resistance or those who must inject insulin.

4. Lower Triglyceride Levels: Triglycerides, a form of blood fat, can be decreased as a result of reduced carbohydrate intake. Increased risk of cardiovascular disease, a major consequence of type 2 diabetes, is linked to elevated triglycerides.

5. Higher HDL Cholesterol: According to some research, diets low in carbohydrates may result in higher HDL cholesterol, sometimes known as "good" cholesterol. A lower risk of heart disease is linked to higher HDL levels.

6. Better Blood Pressure: Cutting back on carbohydrates will help control blood pressure, which is important for cardiovascular health and lowering the risk of complications from diabetes.

7. Lessened appetite and Cravings: A diet that prioritizes wholesome fats and proteins can aid in boosting fullness, which in turn lessens appetite and cravings. Individuals may find it simpler to maintain their diet over time as a result.

8. Individualization: A low-carb diet can be modified to meet specific needs, tastes, and metabolic

reactions. While some people may benefit from a moderately reduced carbohydrate consumption, others may need a very low carbohydrate (ketogenic) regimen.

9. Long-Term Lifestyle Change: Adopting a diet low in carbohydrates can help people properly control their type 2 diabetes while improving their general health and well-being.

Benefits:

1. Increased Insulin Sensitivity: Type 2 diabetes is characterized by insulin resistance, which occurs

when the body's cells stop responding to insulin. A low-carbohydrate diet can improve insulin sensitivity, enabling the body to use insulin to control blood sugar levels more successfully.

2. Lessen Blood Sugar Spikes: Carbohydrate-rich foods, particularly those with a high glycemic index, can result in sharp spikes in blood sugar levels. Diabetes sufferers can achieve more stable blood sugar levels throughout the day by cutting back on these meals.

3. Supports Glycemic Control: Improving glycemic control is essential for controlling diabetes and lowering the risk of complications connected to the disease. People can maintain healthier blood sugar levels by eating a diet low in carbohydrates.

4. Reduction in Medication Use: Adopting a diet low in carbohydrates may help some persons with type 2 diabetes lessen their reliance on diabetes drugs, such as oral hypoglycemic agents or insulin. This may result in a lower risk of adverse drug reactions and consequences.

5. Better Cardiovascular Health: Triglyceride levels, HDL cholesterol, and blood pressure are just a few of the cardiovascular risk factors that can be improved with a diet low in carbohydrates. Heart disease is a major consequence among diabetics that might be decreased by lowering these risk factors.

6. Weight Loss and Management: Diets low in carbohydrates frequently result in weight loss, which is advantageous for type 2 diabetics who are overweight or obese. Glycemic management and

insulin sensitivity are enhanced by weight loss.

7. Sustainable Lifestyle Change: Unlike fad diets, a low-carb diet may be maintained over time since it emphasizes full, healthful meals and doesn't call for drastic calorie restriction. This encourages a lifelong transformation as opposed to a quick fix diet.

Principles:

1. Carbohydrate Awareness: Being aware of the amount of carbohydrates in meals is the cornerstone of a diet low in

carbohydrates. This includes choosing complete, unprocessed meals with reduced carbohydrate contents and being aware of the distinction between simple and complex carbohydrates.

2. Put an emphasis on nutrient-dense foods: Place a focus on nutrient-dense foods that are high in fiber, vitamins, and minerals. These consist of leafy greens, berries, nuts, seeds, lean proteins, non-starchy veggies, lean proteins, and healthy fats.

3. Limit Sugary meals: Sugary meals and drinks, including

sweetened drinks, sugary cereals, and candies, should be consumed in moderation or not at all. These can result in sharp blood sugar rises and exacerbate insulin resistance.

4. Select Whole Grains: When choosing grains, go for whole grains like quinoa, brown rice, and oats rather than processed grains because they are higher in fiber and minerals.

5. Watch Portion Sizes: While calorie monitoring is not always required for a diet low in carbohydrates, portion control is

crucial for controlling blood sugar levels and achieving weight goals.

6. Maintain Hydration: Water consumption is important for general health and can help control blood sugar levels. Drinking too much alcohol and sugary beverages can both affect how your blood sugar is managed.

7. Individualization: The amount of carbohydrates consumed should be tailored to each person's demands, metabolic responses, and health objectives. The diet can be modified to meet individual needs

with the assistance of a trained dietician or healthcare professional.

8. Regularly Check Blood Sugar Levels: Checking blood sugar levels on a regular basis helps track the effects of dietary changes and ensures that levels are within goal limits.

It's crucial to keep in mind that each person may react differently to dietary changes, and not every person with type 2 diabetes will react the same way to a diet low in carbohydrates. Therefore, developing a safe and successful dietary plan that is suited to each individual's needs requires close collaboration with a healthcare professional or a certified dietitian with experience in diabetes management. Additionally, for optimal type 2 diabetes management, lifestyle modifications including frequent exercise and stress reduction should be combined with a diet low in carbohydrates.

Chapter 13

Alternate-day fasting

A nutritional strategy known as intermittent fasting cycles between periods of eating and fasting. It has become more well-known as a potential method of controlling type 2 diabetes. Intermittent fasting, when practiced properly and in conjunction with medical supervision, can help people with type 2 diabetes in a number of ways:

1. Increased Insulin Sensitivity: It has been demonstrated that intermittent fasting increases insulin sensitivity, enabling the body to use insulin more efficiently and better control blood sugar levels. For those with insulin resistance, a frequent feature of type 2 diabetes, this may be very helpful.

2. Weight Loss and Weight Management: Type 2 diabetes must be managed by keeping a healthy weight, which intermittent fasting can help with. Weight loss can improve glycemic management and lessen insulin resistance.

3. Lower Blood Sugar Levels: Intermittent fasting can result in more stable blood sugar levels and less blood sugar rises after meals by minimizing the eating window and carbohydrate intake during fasting periods.

4. Increased Fat Burning: The body uses fat reserves as an energy

source when fasting. This may result in less fat building up in tissues, such as the liver, which is important for those who have type 2 diabetes and may also have fatty liver disease.

5. Improved Lipid Profile: Intermittent fasting may have a good impact on triglyceride and cholesterol levels, lowering the risk of cardiovascular problems, which are more frequent among diabetics.

6. Anti-inflammatory benefits: According to certain research, intermittent fasting may have anti-inflammatory benefits that enhance

insulin sensitivity and metabolic health in general.

7. Easier Meal Planning: Because intermittent fasting limits the number of meals consumed each day, it can be easier for some people to schedule their meals. This may encourage more thoughtful food selections and possibly discourage unhealthy snacking.

It's crucial to keep in mind that intermittent fasting may not be suited for everyone, particularly for some populations, such as women who are pregnant or nursing, those who have a history of eating disorders, or those who have other medical concerns. Additionally, those who are elderly or underweight should attempt intermittent fasting cautiously.

In order to effectively control type 2 diabetes with intermittent fasting, it is necessary to:

1. Speak with a Healthcare Professional: Before beginning intermittent fasting, talk with a healthcare professional or a registered dietitian with experience in diabetes management about your objectives. They can advise you on how to use intermittent fasting

safely and assist in determining whether it is appropriate for you.

2. Customize the Approach: Individual needs and tastes should be taken into consideration while determining the fasting length and eating window. Finding a fasting plan that can be maintained over time and is manageable is crucial.

3. Check Blood Sugar Levels: During intermittent fasting, check blood sugar levels frequently to make sure it isn't having a negative impact on glycemic control.

4. Maintain Hydration: To maintain hydration during fasting, drink lots of water and steer clear of drinks with a lot of caffeine or sugar.

5. Monitor for Hypoglycemia: Be aware of the possibility of hypoglycemia (low blood sugar) during fasting periods if you're taking diabetic drugs, especially if you're taking insulin or sulfonylureas.

6. Put an Emphasis on Nutrient-Dense Foods: When eating, give priority to foods that are high in nutrients and support general health.

In order to effectively manage type 2 diabetes, intermittent fasting must be used carefully and under a doctor's supervision. It does not take the place of other crucial elements of managing diabetes, like medication adherence, consistent exercise, and lifestyle changes.

Chapter 14

Long meal plan

A healthy, balanced diet for someone with type 2 diabetes should include plenty of lean protein, non-starchy vegetables, healthy fats, and whole grains. Avoiding processed foods, refined grains, and sugary drinks is also important. Some good meal ideas for a person with type 2 diabetes include things like chicken and vegetables with a whole grain side, oatmeal with fruit, or a salad with salmon. It's also important to focus on portion control and make sure to eat a consistent amount of food throughout the day.

Examples

Lean protein

Lean proteins are those that are low in saturated fat. Some good options include skinless chicken or turkey, fish like salmon or tuna, lean cuts of beef or pork, and eggs. Beans, lentils, and tofu are also good plant-based sources of protein.

It's important to choose these foods that are prepared without a lot of added fat or sodium. For example, baked or grilled chicken instead of fried chicken, or grilled fish instead of fish with a cream sauce. These are just a few examples, but there are many more options to choose from.

Non starchy vegetables

Non-starchy vegetables are those that have a low glycemic index, meaning they won't cause a large spike in blood sugar. Some examples include leafy greens like spinach or kale, broccoli, cauliflower, asparagus, bell peppers, brussels sprouts, and carrots.

These vegetables can be eaten raw, steamed, sauteed, or roasted, and they can be added to salads, soups, or casseroles. They are a great source of vitamins, minerals, and fiber, and they are low in calories.

Healthy fat

Healthy fats are those that are unsaturated and contain omega-3 fatty acids. Some good sources include olive oil, avocados, nuts like almonds or walnuts, and seeds like chia or flaxseed. These fats can be used in cooking, as salad dressings, or just eaten as a snack. They can help lower cholesterol and improve heart health.

It's important to limit saturated fats found in animal products like butter, full-fat dairy, and fatty meats. Trans fats found in processed foods like cookies or doughnuts should also be avoided.

Whole grain

Whole grains are those that contain the entire grain kernel, including the bran, germ, and endosperm. They are a good source of fiber, protein, and other nutrients. Some examples of whole grains include whole wheat, brown rice, quinoa, oats, barley, and farro.

These can be used in place of refined grains like white bread or pasta.

They can be used in many recipes, including stews, salads, or even as a side dish. It's important to choose whole grains that are not processed with added sugars, like some cereals or breakfast bars.